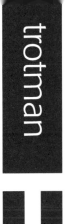

trotman

Real
Life
GUIDES

CARE

Emma Caprez

Real Life Guide to Care

This first edition published in 2006 by Trotman and Company Ltd
2 The Green, Richmond, Surrey TW9 1PL

Editorial and Publishing Team

Author Emma Caprez

Editorial Mina Patria, Editorial Director; Jo Jacomb, Editorial Manager; Catherine Travers, Managing Editor; Ian Turner, Editorial Assistant

Production Ken Ruskin, Head of Pre-press and Production; James Rudge, Production Artworker

Sales and Marketing Suzanne Johnson, Marketing Manager

Advertising Tom Lee, Commercial Director

Design by XAB

British Library Cataloguing in Publications Data

A catalogue record for this book is available from the British Library

ISBN 1 84455 107 5

Typeset by Photoprint, Torquay
Printed and bound in Great Britain
by Creative Print & Design Group, Wales

Real Life GUIDES

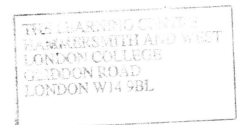

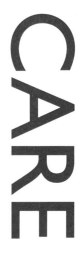

CARE

REAL LIFE GUIDES

Practical guides for practical people

In this increasingly sophisticated world the need for manually skilled people to build our homes, cut our hair, fix our boilers and to make our cars go is greater than ever. As things progress, so the level of training and competence required of our skilled manual workers increases.

In this series of career guides from Trotman, we look in detail at what it takes to train for, get into, and be successful at a wide spectrum of practical careers. The *Real Life Guides* aim to inform and inspire young people and adults alike by providing comprehensive yet hard-hitting and often blunt information about what it takes to succeed in these careers.

Other titles in the series are:

Real Life Guide: The Armed Forces
Real Life Guide: The Beauty Industry
Real Life Guide: Carpentry and Cabinet-Making
Real Life Guide: Catering
Real Life Guide: Construction
Real Life Guide: Distribution and Logistics
Real Life Guide: Electrician
Real Life Guide: The Fire Service
Real Life Guide: Hairdressing
Real Life Guide: The Motor Industry
Real Life Guide: The Police Force
Real Life Guide: Plumbing
Real Life Guide: Retailing
Real Life Guide: Transport
Real Life Guide: Working Outdoors
Real Life Guide: Working with Animals and Wildlife
Real Life Guide: Working with Young People

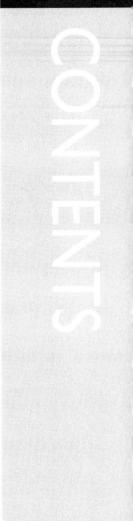

About the author

Emma Caprez has written for various music publications and university literature. For Trotman Publishing she has written *Getting into the Media, Getting into the Performing Arts, Journalism Uncovered, Art and Design Uncovered, The Disabled Students' Guide to University* and *Real Life Issues: Bullying*. She has also written *Tommy's Dad*, a children's book for Action for Prisoners' Families illustrated by Nick Sharratt. She lives in London with her husband, Rook, and two children, BibaMaya and Suky-Ella.

Acknowledgements

I would like to thank the following people for contributing towards this book:

Lynn Towers
Gerry Buckley
Paula Armfield
Laura Towers
Ian Pitchford
Jess Parker

And of course, I would also like to thank my lovely family, Rook, BibaMaya, Suky-Ella, and the rest of my family – Arlette, Dicky, Peach, Timo and Maisie, Lynn, John – and my very caring friends; you know who you are.

Foreword

A career in Care, be it paid or unpaid, is one of the most rewarding and important opportunities available to young people today. Everyone at some stage of their life requires care from others, and at every stage, people have the right to be treated as individuals and receive the best possible quality of support and assistance, delivered with dignity and respect.

To guarantee that individuals receive this quality of care, the Care industry is regulated with a great deal of emphasis placed on the learning and development of those working in this sector. For workers and learners to achieve the required knowledge and standards, and to prove competence, City & Guilds, working with sector skills councils and regulatory bodies, have developed qualifications to help raise standards.

City & Guilds has always been a major provider of qualifications (award 71% of Care related NVQs) in the care sector. We work closely with many important organisations such the NSPCC, Carers UK, NHS, and the Mental Health Foundation to mention just a few. This level of involvement in the Care sector enables us to deliver some of the most up-to-date, relevant and flexible qualifications, which suit learners of all levels, with high levels of recognition from employers throughout the UK.

Our qualifications support learners from pre entry to employment, including modern apprenticeships, with progression right through to management, professional or further education. We have assessment methods to suit all learning styles, ranging from up to the minute e-learning, to the more traditional work placed assessment (N/SVQs) or college based assignment work (VRQs).

Some of our major qualifications, which can form part of modern apprenticeships, include N/SVQs in Health and Social Care, Health and Children's Care, Learning and Development. In these areas we also offer vocationally related qualifications (VRQs) which develop knowledge and understanding, and these can be used to assist entry or progression. Some of these VRQs include work in specialist areas like mental health and learning disabilities.

City & Guilds are delighted to be part of the Trotman Real Life Guides series to help raise your awareness of these vocational qualifications. If the opportunity of involvement in Care appeals to you, City & Guilds has qualifications which will support development throughout your career, helping you to achieve excellence and quality in whatever field you choose.

Introduction

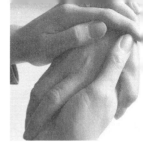

WHAT IS CARE WORK?

Social care and social work are about helping improve people's quality of life. Those you care for may be vulnerable, lonely or disadvantaged in some way and may feel excluded or undervalued by society. Care is all about building relationships with these people and offering practical support so that they can cope with their everyday lives.

WHAT'S THE DIFFERENCE BETWEEN SOCIAL CARE AND SOCIAL WORK?

Social care: People working in social work offer personal care to a variety of people in residential homes, in their own homes, at day centres and in schools. You can start a social care job without qualifications, but you will be expected to undergo training to gain skills and qualifications that will be updated on a regular basis.

Social work: Social workers assess individual care needs and work with other organisations (such as care homes, hospitals and the police service) to ensure support needs are met. They are registered professionals who have gained a recognised degree in social work.

MAKING A DIFFERENCE

How we care for the more vulnerable people in our society is a reflection of how we are as a nation. Everyone deserves to be treated with dignity and respect – especially those who really need our support. Helping someone to achieve their individual needs, and seeing their face light up as a result, is a real reward for people in the care sector. Without the right assistance, many people will not have the quality of life and the dignity they deserve.

How we care for the more vulnerable people in our society is a reflection of how we are as a nation.

Care is all about enabling people to cope with their daily lives – whether by helping them with their shopping, helping them to communicate or helping them fit into life in a new country. When it's time for you to put your feet up at the end of a busy day (or night!), you can be happy that you've made an important difference to someone's life.

A STEREOTYPICAL CARER?

If you think about working in care, what images come to mind? Do you see a middle-aged female carer looking after an elderly client, perhaps in a care home or perhaps in their own home? That's the stereotype – but although there are undoubtedly plenty of carers who correspond with this image, in reality the sector is much more varied.

For a start, care workers are drawn from a range of age groups (see box on page 3). And then there is the fact that looking after the elderly is not the only care work available (although it is of course a very important job). As a care worker you could work with people from any age group in any location – for example, you could be a personal assistant caring for a child with a disability in their own home, or you could work in the community to support adults with mental health difficulties or families experiencing problems. The care sector also extends to supporting people who are not vulnerable, but who just want a bit of extra help – for example with childcare, gardening or cleaning.

The one stereotype that does, for the moment at least, ring true, is that the care workforce is overwhelmingly female – according to the Office for National Statistics, 88% of care workers are women. This is partly because, rightly or wrongly, the role of caring for people still tends to be seen by society as a feminine one. However, the sector is developing fast and is keen to attract both male and female workers, so there is no reason to believe that the all-female stereotype will still ring true in the future. Care is a growing industry with good training prospects, flexible work options and better opportunities to develop your career than ever before.

AGE PROFILE OF THE CARE WORKFORCE
- 16% are aged 24 years or under
- 20% are aged between 25 and 34
- 39% are aged between 35 and 49
- 25% are aged over 50

Source: Office for National Statistics

AN INCREASINGLY IMPORTANT JOB

Care is increasingly becoming recognised as an extremely important job sector. In early 2006, the Department of Health launched a national recruitment campaign to highlight the importance of care work in our communities and to encourage people of all ages and backgrounds to consider choosing this career option. You can check out the campaign websites for yourself on www.socialcarecareers.co.uk and www.socialworkcareers.co.uk.

The growing importance of caring roles has also been reflected in the move to professionalise the sector. In the past, care workers did not need any formal qualifications, but now they are required to develop and advance their skills by taking nationally recognised qualifications. This doesn't mean that you necessarily need to have these qualifications before starting a job in care (you can train while you work) – but it does mean you will be given the opportunity to learn and to gain professional recognition for the work you do. (See Chapter 7 for more detailed information on training.)

IS THERE A JOB IN CARE FOR ME?

It doesn't matter what your age is or whether you have any qualifications – the care sector is enormous, with a broad

DID YOU KNOW?

The social care and health industry is currently one of the largest employers in the country – and the need for it is ever-increasing. An estimated two million contacts from new clients were made to councils with Social Service Responsibilities (SSRs) in England in the year 2004–5.

Source: Community Care Statistics 2004–05: Referrals, Assessments and Packages of Care for Adults, England: National Summary

range of jobs available offering challenge, variety and rewards. What's more, promotion prospects are good: the sector is growing, so care workers are needed to take responsibility for organising staffing, services and training.

HOW THIS BOOK WILL HELP

If you enjoy working with people and want to make a difference to someone's life, then a job in the care sector could be right up your street – this book will help you decide whether care is for you and, if it is, help you find out more about which kinds of job interest you the most. The first four chapters give you a broad overview of the sector and the kind of work you might be doing; then the second part of the book helps you focus in on whether you have the skills and personality to succeed in the sector, and what training and career routes are available to you.

FAST FACTS ON CARE

A survey was carried out in September 2005 to investigate the amount and nature of care services taking place during one week. It revealed that:

- An estimated 3.6 million contact hours were provided to around 354,500 households (or 367,700 clients)
- The average number of contact hours per household was 10.1 hours per week
- 15% of households receiving care had only a single visit during the week

- Around 98,200 households (28% of the total) received intensive home care in 2005 (defined as more than 10 hours and 6 or more visits during the week).

Source: Community Care Statistics 2005: Home Help and Care Services for Adults, England, provided by Councils with Social Services Responsibilities (CSSR) for the Department of Health

Statistics available for the year 2004–5 show that:

- There were an estimated 1.72 million clients receiving services during the year
- In respect of waiting times for new clients ages 65 and over, about 26% of all new older clients had their assessment completed within 2 days of first contact and 55% were assessed within 2 weeks, an increase on the previous year, but below ministerial target of 70%.

Source: Community Care Statistics 2004–05: Referrals, Assessments and Packages of Care for Adults, England: National Summary

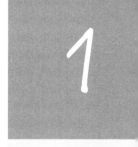

IAN PITCHFORD

Success story

COMMUNITY MENTAL HEALTH NURSE

Ian Pitchford is a community mental health nurse for the South Camden Crisis Response and Resolution team based at St Pancras Hospital, part of Camden and Islington Social Care Trust.

'My job involves assessing mental health and risk in relation to clients receiving home treatment – this is usually an alternative to admitting them to hospital. I assess social needs and make referrals to other services where necessary, and I do link work with local A&E (accident and emergency) departments, GP practices and community mental health needs. I also provide home treatment, which involves giving one-to-one support, monitoring and administering medication and making psychological interventions [for example by providing counselling]. I am an active member of a multi-disciplinary team, including supervising staff and training.

'I am a Registered Mental Health Nurse (Project 2000 – diploma level training) and I have regular training updates. For my job I needed to have had a minimum of one year's experience working with acutely

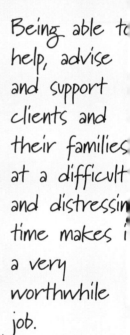

Being able to help, advise and support clients and their families at a difficult and distressin time makes i a very worthwhile job.

It's important to be able to solve problems, to have organisational skills and to be able to use intervention techniques.

unwell clients or Community Mental Health Team (CMHT) experience. At the level I practice you've already passed through lower nursing grades. Skills include communicating with clients, family members and other professionals. It's important to be able to solve problems, to have organisational skills and to be able to use intervention techniques.

'The pros of my job are being able to support clients in their own homes, to reinforce the clients' coping skills and to avoid hospital admissions, often when other professionals feel this is not possible. Treating clients in their own environments enables you to reinforce the personal responsibilities which are often removed by the hospital system. I also like to feel part of the client's community via the social systems approach. I get more money for working unsocial hours – we offer a 24-hour service. Being able to help, advise and support clients and their families at a difficult and distressing time makes it a very worthwhile job.

'The cons are inappropriate referrals – I often feel that, due to the accessibility of the service, we get referrals as a result of the failures of other services because of inaction. There's also stress caused by decision-making and positive risk taking. We work on an on-call rota so I can work strange hours. Again, because of the accessibility of our service I often have to deal with the frustration of referrals and clients and their families – generally not because of our actions, but because of politics, lack of funding and cutbacks.'

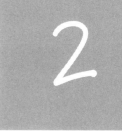

Would you care to know?

What will the work be like? Who might you work for – and with? What are the entry requirements? This chapter answers these and other questions you might have about working in care.

WHO WILL I WORK FOR?
Possible employers might include:

- Local authorities
- Health authorities
- Private organisations and agencies
- Voluntary organisations
- The church
- Charities
- Individuals.

WHERE WILL I WORK?
Care work takes place in a variety of environments, including:

- Private homes
- Hospitals (NHS and private)
- Residential and nursing care homes
- Prisons
- Schools
- Community centres

- Youth clubs
- Drop-in centres
- Council offices.

WHO WILL MY CLIENTS BE?

As a care worker you will be helping people who, for whatever reason, need your support. These people can be of any age and from any walk of life. Groups of people who may be in particular need of support may include:

- People with physical and/or learning disabilities
- People with mental health issues
- People who are ill – both short-term and long-term
- Older people
- People displaying antisocial behaviour
- Drug addicts
- Offenders
- Families facing a variety of issues
- Minority ethnic groups
- Refugees and asylum seekers
- Travellers
- People who are homeless
- People who are at risk of sexual exploitation
- People who just want extra help coping with their lives.

WHO WILL MY COLLEAGUES BE?

You will be part of a team working closely with many other agencies and organisations in order to cater for your clients' needs. For example, you may work with:

AGENCY WORK

Agencies provide care work to other organisations – so instead of being employed by, for example, a health authority, you might be employed by an agency to do work for a health authority. There are numerous agencies spread throughout the country, some specialising in providing workers of a certain type (for example social workers or occupational therapists) and others providing staff across the whole sector.

Agency work is generally better paid and often incentives such as golden hellos will be offered, but you do need to be wary about being thrown into a job that you are not necessarily experienced to do, especially as you may not have the support you require from colleagues. You will also need to organise your own private pension.

Another important factor to consider with agency work is training. The General Social Care Council's registration requirement for social workers is that 90 hours of post-qualifying training must be completed within three years. If you work for an agency, you may have to foot the training bill yourself.

- Health professionals such as clinical psychologists, physiotherapists and specialist nurses
- Council departments
- Social services
- Housing providers
- The police service

DID YOU KNOW?

Those who you support are referred to as your clients. The word 'client' comes from the Latin cluere meaning 'to hear' or 'to obey' — this meaning is still very relevant today, as care workers listen to what their clients have to say, and cater for their needs.

- The courts
- The voluntary sector
- Employment agencies.

Each organisation provides a vital piece of the care jigsaw, and you will all be working together towards the same goal – however, since so many different organisations may be involved, communication and administration can sometime be complicated.

HOW OLD DO I HAVE TO BE?

Some posts in care are open to young people aged 16 years and over, while for others you will need to be a minimum of 18 years old. The Commission for Social Care Inspection has developed national minimum standards which include requirements regarding the employment and supervision of young people.

WILL I HAVE PRE-EMPLOYMENT CHECKS?

Pre-employment checks are a necessity in this area of work – you will be in a position where you are responsible for the welfare of vulnerable people and it is therefore vital that your employers can check that you do not have criminal

Each organisation provides a vital piece of the care jigsaw, and you will all be working together towards the same goal.

convictions that might suggest you are not suitable for this kind of work.

You will be asked to provide references and to undergo a **Criminal Records Bureau (CRB)** check – for more information on this, see www.crb.gov.uk. If you plan to work with adults, you will be checked against the **Protection of Vulnerable Adults (POVA)** list to determine if you have previously harmed vulnerable adults. If you plan to work with children under the age of 18 you will be checked against the **Protection of Children Act (PoCA)** list.

WHAT QUALIFICATIONS DO I NEED?

You can enter many care jobs with no qualifications, and you will be offered on-the-job training towards nationally-recognised qualifications. However, for some of the more specialised jobs (such as social worker or occupational therapist) you may need an NVQ, diploma or even a degree. Qualifications and entry to the sector is dealt with in-depth in Chapter 7.

WHAT ARE THE WORKING CONDITIONS LIKE?

Many jobs in care offer flexible working hours, which is great if you don't want to work the normal nine-to-five routine or you need something that will fit around your other commitments (such as part-time education courses or family). Depending on the work, you may be required to work some antisocial hours and night shifts.

DID YOU KNOW?

In 2004, the average gross annual pay across the care workforce was £11,004, and the average gross hourly pay was £6.73.

Source: Office for National Statistics

You may be travelling around a lot, so it can also be useful (and it is sometimes a requirement) to have a driving licence and to own a car. Some care positions include live-in accommodation (especially in areas where it is more expensive to live) – however, this is less common than it used to be.

The care sector is not renowned for its high wages. People tend to do the job because they find it rewarding rather than for the money – although if you are ambitious and work your way up to more senior positions, the financial rewards can be impressive. More detailed information on salaries is given in the next chapter.

WHERE DO I LOOK FOR WORK?

Care workers are always needed. Check out the following places to find jobs advertised:

- Local newspaper
- Local council website
- Websites and publications
- Job centre.

Check the Resources chapter at the end of this book for further information.

Who cares?

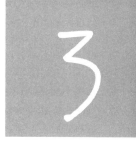

The previous chapters should have given you a good overview of what the care sector is all about – now it's time to get down to the nitty-gritty details. From residential care to occupational therapy, the range of jobs in the care sector is immense – where do you start? What jobs are available? What sort of tasks might you actually be carrying out? How much might you earn?

This chapter outlines the type of work involved in a variety of positions and gives an indication of the kind of salary you might receive. Pay is, of course, dependent on a number of factors (for example the nature of the job and the geographical area you are working in). Each employing organisation will negotiate their own salaries within certain guidelines. All salaries stated in this chapter are therefore intended as a guide only.

HOME CARE
There are two reasons why people may require care within their own homes:

1) Because of need (eg disability or illness)
2) Because they just desire extra help.

HOME CARE BECAUSE OF NEED
If you become a **home care assistant** or **home care worker** you will work as part of a team to provide practical support and regular human contact in order to enable vulnerable people to remain living at home. For people living

on their own (especially older people), you may be the only person that they see on a regular basis, so you will be providing both social and emotional support.

DID YOU KNOW?

39% of those aged over 65 receiving home care said their care workers 'always' or 'usually' came at convenient times, and 65% said changes were always made when requested.

Source: Personal Social Services: Survey of home care users in England aged 65 or over, 2002–3

You will need to be aware of each client's circumstances and listen and respond to their individual needs. A home care worker's role could include:

- Personal care (eg help with washing, dressing and household tasks)
- Shopping
- Help with administrative tasks (eg sorting out benefits, paying bills)
- Keeping an eye on the client's health issues (eg ensuring doctors' appointments are made, pills are taken, etc).

Home care assistants and care workers can expect to earn in the region of £10,000–£13,000 per year, or be paid at a rate of £5–£9 per hour. Senior care assistants can earn around £18,000–£20,000 per year.

HOME CARE FOR THOSE WHO WANT EXTRA HELP
Some people just lead hectic lives and need extra help around the home. Others choose to bring in help in order to free up more of their own time for leisure pursuits. This help could be in the form of gardening, cleaning or looking after their children, and it will not be dealt with in detail in this book – see *Real Life Guides: Working with Young People* for

more information on nannying and other childcare roles, and *Real Life Guides: Working Outdoors* for more information on gardening.

Gardeners, cleaners and childminders are often self-employed and charge their clients an hourly rate – for domestic cleaners and childminders, these may start at around £5 per hour; gardeners and garden designers may charge a little more, depending on their experience.

CLOSE-UP ON NANNYING

If you become a nanny you will support parents by looking after their children. Some nannies are employed from a child's birth to help with the demands of a newborn baby, including getting up in the night to feed and change the baby. The job of a nanny may involve many different tasks depending on the parents' wishes; things you might be asked to do for the children you look after include:

- Cooking
- Feeding
- Bathing
- Helping get dressed
- Taking to and from school
- Helping with homework
- Organising social life (eg having other children round to play and taking the children out to the playground and other outings).

Qualifications are not essential, but they are definitely becoming preferable. Salaries vary depending on geographical location, level of qualifications and whether you are employed by an agency or by the family. Full-time nannies can earn anything from £9,000–£18,000+.

RESIDENTIAL CARE

For a variety of reasons, some people are unable to cope with living at home. It is the job of **residential care workers** to ensure that these people are treated with dignity in an environment that ensures they are safe, clean and comfortable and to bring happiness and company to their lives.

Residential care homes usually specialise in providing support for a particular group of people – for example, children being looked after, adults with special needs or the elderly, who are no longer able to live in their own homes. You need to be able to build relationships with these people, to gain their trust and see to their needs. Depending on the nature of your clients, you may help them deal with issues that might be of concern to them (for example low self-esteem or problems faced at school and puberty), and you may help them develop more practical skills such as cooking and looking after their finances.

If you work in residential care, you may become a **key worker**, working with a resident on a one-to-one basis, supporting them with their leisure pursuits and escorting them on trips outside of the

DID YOU KNOW?

According to the Office for National Statistics, there are currently 549,000 care assistants and home carers in the care workforce.

CARING FOR THE ELDERLY

It has recently been highlighted in the media that older people are not always treated with the dignity or respect they deserve in many care homes and hospitals across Britain. This can only be a reflection of the way older people are viewed in society. Of course, the difference between any good or bad care service is dependent on whether the staff are considerate and responsive to the individual needs of their clients. If you can show you care by working in this vitally important profession, you can bring about change, not only to the individuals concerned, but society at large.

A recent survey by the Department of Health entitled 'Dignity in Care' has suggested that frequent staff changes and patronising attitudes were amongst the chief problems, and has suggested the following measures to improve the situation:

- Better pay
- More staff
- Improved training
- More personalised service
- Tougher penalties for failing agencies.

residential home, for example to college or social events. You may need to do nightshifts on a rota basis or be required to live in. It is possible to do this work on a part-time basis to fit around other commitments.

Like home care assistants/workers, residential care workers can expect to earn in the region of £10,000–£13,000 per year, or be paid at a rate of £5–£9 per hour. If you work unsociable hours in a residential centre then your salary could increase to £16,000 a year. Senior care assistants can earn around £18,000–£20,000 per year.

SOCIAL CARE

DAY CARE
Day care assistants enable service users (clients who come and use the services available at the day centres) to integrate with other people, get involved in activities and learn new skills which lead to a better quality of life and greater independence, all within a safe and supportive environment. If you work in day care services you will be responsible for supporting and caring for people with disabilities, mental health issues, older people and people with a range of other issues including young offenders.

Support workers work with individual clients (eg people with alcohol or substance abuse problems) on a one-to-one basis to help them deal with their needs.

Day care assistants and support workers are usually paid approximately £6–£8 per hour, depending on location, hours and experience. For full-time, permanent employees, salaries are usually around £11,000–£13,000, but can rise to £18,000 or over.

INDEPENDENT LIVING
Some people with disabilities need to have the support of a **personal assistant (PA)** to enable them to live their lives

independently. As a PA you will be required to work on a one-to-one basis with your client, supporting them with their individual needs. The support you offer your client will be varied, depending both on the nature of their disability and the choices they make – for example, you may:

- Help your client to get dressed
- Fit prosthetic limbs
- Take notes in university lectures
- Take your client out to social events.

Personal assistants are usually paid a similar wage to day care assistants and support workers (see above).

Communication support workers (CSWs) work with deaf and hard-of-hearing students who are studying at further or higher education colleges and universities. If you work in this area you will be responsible for ensuring that your client is as able to gain the same information as everyone else on their course. This will be achieved by the use of a range of methods depending on your client's needs – these could include

- British Sign Language
- Note-taking
- Lipspeaking.

DID YOU KNOW?

46% of those receiving social services support for their disabilities were 'extremely satisfied' or 'very satisfied' with the help they received. However, only 29% said that their opinions and preferences were always taken into account when decisions were taken about the services provided to them.

Source: Personal Social Services: Survey of physically disabled and sensory impaired users in England aged 18–64, 2003–4

The work you undertake will depend on your skills and qualifications. You may be employed directly by the educational establishment your clients attend, or by a freelance agency. Your work is likely to be part time and within academic terms, and you will be part of a team including the teaching staff at the institute at which your client is learning and other professionals as necessary.

If you are ambitious, you may be able to move into more senior positions, in which you will be responsible for coordinating a team of CSWs. Experienced CSWs could also move into teaching, either of British Sign Language or for people who are deaf or hard of hearing.

Unqualified communication support workers can earn around £12,000–£14,000 per year. With qualifications and experience this can rise to £15,500–£20,000.

FIELDWORK WITH ADULTS

Fieldworkers work with people who need extra help to cope with everyday life – for example those with mental health issues or learning disabilities or those who are refugees. This means going out and making contact with the people who need support, building relationships with them and gaining their trust, then helping them overcome any barriers or problems they face (for example, language barriers).

DID YOU KNOW?

Community-based services were provided to about 1.47 million clients during the year 2004–5, accounting for 85% of all clients receiving services.

Source: Community Care Statistics 2004–05: Referrals, Assessments and Packages of Care for Adults, England: National Summary

You may become a community **outreach worker**, whose main concern is making people aware of their entitlements and rights, so that they do not become marginalised. Ensuring people are aware of the services that are available to them, such as healthcare and day centres, means that people can make informed choices.

You will need to be able to present and push forward your clients' views to other social care/health staff, and to be able to negotiate with service providers on your clients' behalf. You may have to accompany or represent service users at case conferences or tribunals.

Fieldwork also extends to young people who are finding life difficult to cope with. These young people may have substance abuse or behavioural problems which include illegal activities. **Youth workers** help young people find a way out of their problems by encouraging their social, personal and educational development – this work can take place at clubs or centres or, more informally, in shopping centres or on the street.

Fieldworkers are usually paid approximately £6–£8 per hour, depending on location, hours and experience. For full-time, permanent employees, salaries are usually around £11,000–£13,000, but can rise to £18,000 or over. A mental health outreach worker employed by local government might earn £12,500–£15,500 per year. A qualified youth worker can earn £15,000–£18,000, rising to £20,000–£25,000 with experience. Senior workers can earn £30,000 plus.

Family support workers work with families at times of crisis. These families will be referred to you by a social worker, and may be experiencing problems with parenting, violence, deprivation or drug misuse. You will be supporting the parents and helping them to gain skills such as:

- Dealing with the emotional and social welfare of their children (including discipline)
- Managing the home (for example domestic chores and cleanliness)
- Managing their financial affairs (for example budgeting, bill paying etc).

You will need to write up reports of the cases you are working on and you may be required to provide evidence in court if there is a care order taken out on the children you are working with. Sometimes, it may be necessary to go and live in the family home when the children need to be cared for due to the absence of their parent(s). This will just be a short-term measure until alternatives are sought, but it can happen if, for example, a parent is taken into hospital, sent to prison or abandons their child.

You will work with a social worker and your manager to plan the kind of care requirements that are needed and how long they will be needed for. On-the-job training will include child protection, first aid and recognising drug and alcohol abuse as well as family assessment.

Family support workers typically earn around £14,000–£16,000 per year. With experience this can rise to £19,000–£25,000 per year.

SOCIAL WORK

SOCIAL WORK ASSISTANTS

Social work assistants support social workers in all their daily responsibilities (see below). If you become a social work assistant you will need to carry out administrative duties such as:

- Contacting clients and arranging appointments
- Dealing with enquiries
- Organising and taking part in meetings with the social work team and the other agencies involved
- Making needs assessments for clients.

Like social workers, social work assistants work in a variety of places including hospitals, hostels, residential care homes, day care centres and the community. They earn around £14,000–£15,000 per year, rising to £21,000 with experience and the relevant NVQs.

SOCIAL WORKERS

As a social worker you will work with vulnerable people, assess their needs and deliver solutions for their care requirements. This might involve helping clients to sort out housing, health issues or benefits. You may work with a wide range of people such as children, older people, people with mental health issues, people with disabilities or illness such as HIV/AIDs. You will also work with your clients' family and friends.

You will write reports on the clients you are working with and these will be required by a certain deadline. You will be responsible for compiling care plans with an agenda of goals

DID YOU KNOW?

According to the Office for National Statistics, there are currently 79,000 social workers in the UK.

and what you hope to achieve. Sometimes, things go wrong and it is extremely important that you are able to assess the level of risk to those involved and act accordingly.

You will work closely with and liaise between the different agencies involved, such as teachers and doctors. You may be responsible for recruiting, supporting and delivering training to other members of staff as well as arranging foster parents for children and young people in care. Raising awareness of the field you are working in to other professionals and reducing stigma will be another element to your work. You may also teach students who are in their final year of their social work degree.

Your work may include nightshifts on a rota basis, and residential social workers will probably be required to work some weekends. Social workers can be self-employed. There are two types of social worker:

1. **Residential social worker** – works with people living in residential homes (residential social workers may also be known as care officers or residential support workers)
2. **Field social worker** – works within the community or other settings, such as in healthcare.

The starting salary for a probationary or newly-qualified social worker is around £15,000–£17,000 per annum; with experience this can rise to £18,000–£32,000 per year or £12 to £23 an hour. Field social workers can earn

£18,000–£30,000 dependent on experience and specialist skills. Senior residential social workers will earn in the region of £28,000–£45,000.

Social workers can choose to specialise in a range of areas, including:

- Community care
- Offenders
- Mental health
- Children and families
- HIV/AIDS.

Each area involves specialist work. For example, if you choose to specialise in working with children and families, you might:

- Work with at-risk children who need protecting
- Arrange fostering or adoption of children whose families are unable to care for them safely
- Help parents who are having difficulties coping with their children

---

SOCIAL CARE REGISTER

Social Workers, qualified or student, who operate in England, must now join the General Social Care Council's Social Care Register. This register is a new development and means that you must abide by the General Social Care Council's Code of Practice for Social Care Workers. This register will soon be open to other social care workers.

- Support young adults who are leaving care so that they can live independently
- Try to keep families together.

Social workers can progress to a wide variety of career areas such as management, teaching and consultancy. **Senior social workers** will have added financial, administrative and supervisory responsibilities.

MANAGERIAL POSITIONS

As outlined in the introduction to this book, the care sector is growing fast and this means that more senior, managerial positions are becoming available to those who can prove they have the skills and experience to take them on. These positions vary hugely – from taking responsibility for one or two members of staff as part of a bigger agency to running your own care home or developing care strategy at a high level.

After a few years' experience, you may find you can apply for positions involving:

- Managing staff
- Ensuring that staff are properly trained
- Organising rotas or shifts
- Keeping up-to-date with research, inquiries and inspections
- Contributing ideas, problem solving and negotiation.

Of course, bureaucracy and red-tape is involved and lots of paperwork can be time-consuming. More senior management positions involve bringing about change for the better regarding the way things are run in your organisation and for the clients you serve, by:

- Developing partnerships with other services that are relevant to your work (such as the health and police services)
- Setting up advisory groups
- Inspecting care homes and writing inspection reports
- Gathering feedback and reviewing progress to ensure that needs are being met, funding is coming in and projects are initiated and budgeted for
- Marketing and promoting of the field of work you are in.

You may need further qualifications and strategic/management experience in order to secure this kind of job. Care managers might earn in the region of £20,000–£40,000 per year depending on the nature of their work. Project coordinators could earn around £35,000 and at senior level you can earn from £38,000 to £60,000+.

If you become a **care home manager** you will be required to meet the National Minimum Standards as laid out in health care legislation issued by the Department of Health. These standards will vary according to the client group your care home is providing a service for. A job of this nature will require some nightshift work and working at weekends and you may have to live in.

OTHER JOBS IN CARE

OCCUPATIONAL THERAPY

Occupational Therapists (OTs) work with people who have disabilities so that they can remain at home and live independently. Work involves visiting clients in their own homes, assessing their needs and ensuring that they receive the advice, information, equipment and adaptations to the property they require in order to live full independent lifestyles. You may also have to assess the client's carer to ensure that they are caring for the client safely. Being an OT requires you to liaise with other workers such as physiotherapists, health professionals and so on. There is a growing trend for occupational therapists being employed in council housing departments.

OTs earn around £18,000–£21,000 per year, and experienced OTs can earn up to £36,000. Senior OTs earn in the region of £42,000–£51,000 per year.

DID YOU KNOW?

According to www.cot.org.uk, 'there are over 26,000 qualified occupational therapists in the UK, working in the NHS, social services, local authorities, independent practice, voluntary agencies, universities and the commercial sector'.

Occuptional Therapy Support Workers (OTSWs) assist OTs in helping cater for clients' needs in order to cope with their daily routine and have a better quality of life. The main part of the OTSWs role is to encourage clients to work towards the targets that they have agreed with the OT. This may be, for example, encouraging a client to learn to talk again after having had a stroke or stimulating a client with mental health issues to take up an art class at a local college. As an OTSW you will need to monitor clients' progress and write up reports which will be delivered to the OT.

You will work in a variety of settings including day centres and residential homes as well as hospitals or in the clients' own homes, and you will earn about £11,000–£13,000 per year, which rises to £14,150 with experience and relevant NVQ qualifications.

COUNSELLING

Counsellors use a range of different methods to help gain their clients' trust, working through issues that may be causing them distress and helping their personal development. There are a number of different counselling methods, including:

- Cognitive
- Humanistic
- Behavioural
- Person-centred.

If you become a counsellor you will work in an environment that enables your client to feel calm and relaxed so that they can explore why they are feeling the way they do and consider how to resolve it. Sometimes, you may have to carry out your counselling over the phone. Opportunities exist for experienced counsellors to move into managerial roles or open up their own practice.

Many people carry out counselling work on a part-time basis alongside another career. They might be paid £30–£50 per hour for their time if they work with private clients, but many offer their services free of charge for charitable organisations. A qualified and experienced full-time counsellor could earn £15,500–£31,000.

WORK IN SCHOOLS

Care work in schools involves working with individual pupils to help them attain their individual learning targets. Jobs of this nature may have a number of titles, for example:

- Teaching assistant
- Special needs classroom assistant
- Learning support assistant
- Support worker
- Non-teaching support staff.

The pupils you work with may have physical and/or learning disabilities or behavioural problems. Working under the teacher's direction, you will carry out a range of tasks depending on your job description and the nature of the pupil's needs. These could include:

- Support with literacy, numeracy and other educational areas
- Support with social interaction
- Support for physical needs.

You will also ensure that the children in your care are safe. You may work in any type of school (including mainstream schools) and your work will fit in with school hours. A special needs teaching assistant will earn about £10,000–£12,000 per year. This increases with experience to between £14,000 and £17,000 per year. Teaching assistant posts are often part-time. A good way to get into a job such as this is to volunteer to work in the school, as experience of working with children is vital.

RELATED WORK AREAS

If you've read through this chapter and like the idea of some aspects of the work, but not others, don't despair! There are a number of related areas that might appeal to you. For example, you could take a job on the more administrative side of the sector – this means you would play an important role in organising care provision, but you may not have direct contact with clients. Alternatively, you could begin by working in care, using it as a foundation to develop skills which would be transferable to any of the jobs listed below, and vice versa.

- Art/music/drama/play therapy
- British Sign Language/English interpreter
- Charity fundraiser
- Psychologist
- Psychoanalyst
- Nursery nurse.

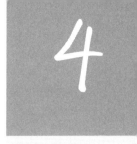

GERRY BUCKLEY

Case study 1

SOCIAL SERVICES OFFICER (SSO)

'I basically do the job of a social worker (SW), but it's not supposed to be like that. I should only really be doing assessments, but I do the whole range. In the past two years I've only ever had one case taken from me and given to an SW, and that was only a minor abuse case – they have left the more serious ones with me for some reason.

'In theory SSOs are only supposed to assess cases and pass them on to an SW, but in practice this is now dying out and we are more involved and are given a lot more responsibility. It boils down to the cheap option, but we are closely monitored by managers and can ask for a case to be reallocated.

'I set up care packages for people over 65 if they are going home, or look for placements if they are not in a position to do this. Placements can be residential, nursing or mental health – I am not an approved social worker (ASW) so I can't section clients.

My advice to someone wishing to do a job like mine would be to make sure it's what you really want to do and then get some experience.

I like the variety of my job. There is also a sense of achievement when a case works out when others are thinking you are barking up the wrong tree.

'I got the job initially because they were very short of staff and I could start the following day! I already had experience of assessments and care packages from 12 years of working with people with learning difficulties and some experience of working with people with mental health issues. What they look for is people who have wide experience and I suppose you have to not be phased by situations and remain professional at all times.

'I like the variety of my job. There is also a sense of achievement when a case works out when others are thinking you are barking up the wrong tree. Personally, I like the hospital side of it as well, because you get to work with staff from a variety of disciplines including consultants, occupational therapists, physios, psychologists – the whole range really.

'The big downside to my job is the amount of paperwork – everybody will mention that as a disadvantage!

'My advice to someone wishing to do a job like mine would be to make sure it's what you really want to do and then get some experience of a variety of client groups before jumping in too deeply.'

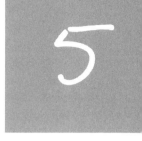

Do you care?

Care work can be extremely rewarding – but on the other hand, it can sometimes be upsetting, stressful and demanding. In order to cope with the physical, mental and emotional demands it makes, you need to be a certain kind of person with skills and abilities to match.

This chapter will explore the general qualities you need to work in the sector, and outline some of the more specific skills you may need for particular jobs. Have a read through and see if you think you fit the bill – then try the quiz on page 41 to help you work out whether you've got what it takes to approach different situations in a caring way.

A CARING PERSONALITY

It may sound obvious, but there's no point in considering a career in the care sector if you're not a caring kind of person. Here are some of the personality traits and skills that you need to make a good carer, together with a brief explanation of why each quality is important. These qualities are required for all jobs in the care sector:

- **An enjoyment of working with people** – because you will be meeting and supporting clients every day – you need to be interested in what they have to say in order to build up a good rapport with them
- **Good communication skills** – because you must be able to communicate effectively both with your clients (to gain their trust and to find out their needs) and with your colleagues (so that they have the information they need to

support you in fulfilling your client's needs; if you are not able to listen to, respond to and cooperate with other team members, the whole system would break down and you would not be able to provide clients with the care they need)

- **Empathy and listening skills** – because it is vitally important that you listen to, understand, sympathise with and respond to the needs of your clients – that's what care work is all about!
- **Respect for others** – because your clients need to know that you value them; this is the basis on which you can build a positive relationship with them
- **Open-mindedness** – because you need to have a non-judgemental attitude towards clients, otherwise you will not be able to gain their trust and get them to open up to you. You need to be able to treat each client as an individual and not make assumptions about them based on their age, physical/mental health, religion or anything else
- **Energy and enthusiasm** – because if you can communicate these emotions to your clients you will build more positive, productive relationships with them
- **Reliability** – because you can't afford to let people down when you are working in care
- **Diplomacy skills** – because you will need to be able to handle complex situations sensitively
- **Patience** – because things won't always go the way you would like them to, and you need to be able to keep calm. (Patience is also particularly useful if you are working with young children!)
- **A well-lined stomach** – because it's no good being squeamish if you plan to work in care; your job may bring you into contact with bodily fluids of all kinds on a regular basis!

- **Resilience and a sense of humour** – because the work can get very tough at times (for example if you are working with a family where there has been a child abuse case, or with a person who becomes seriously ill or even dies) and you need to be able to remain positive and ride the storms.

These qualities will be particularly important for jobs such as care assistant, care worker, support worker and personal assistant, as in these occupations, time spent with the clients is very high and it's possible you may be the main contact with the outside world for some people – that's a big responsibility.

PRACTICAL SKILLS AND QUALITIES

- **Physical fitness** – because you may have to assist your patients by moving or lifting them. If you are a home care worker you may be on your feet for much of the day
- **Good team-work skills** – because you will always work as a team with people from your department and those of other agencies
- **Planning and organisational skills** – because you will be working with other agencies, and planning how you can work together to best help clients progress and cater for their individual needs

- **A knowledge of basic hygiene standards** – this is essential when caring for people who require your support on a personal level. Your initial training (see the next chapter) should teach you what you need to know.

JOB-SPECIFIC SKILLS

COMMUNICATION SUPPORT WORKER

If you want to work with people who have a hearing impairment, you will need to be able to use and understand British Sign Language and/or lipspeaking (as an aid to lipreading). It is also important that you have an awareness and understanding of deaf and blind culture.

SOCIAL WORKERS

Social workers need:

- **The ability to work under pressure and to schedules** – because reports often need to be completed and sometimes quick decisions must be made when, for example, you have to assess the level of risk to a client when things go wrong. Panic and confusion could result in terrible consequences
- **Problem-solving skills and quick thinking** – because you will have to decide how to change people's current quality of life for the best
- **Assessment skills** – because assessing clients' needs is an essential part of your job as a social worker, so aptitude in this area is crucial
- **Advocacy skills** – because your job as a social worker is to support and speak up on the behalf of your clients to help make sure that their needs are catered for.

MANAGERIAL POSITIONS

The following are general skills necessary for most managerial positions, and also for social workers:

- **Project and people management skills** – because you need to be able to get the best out of your team and to maintain a cohesive unit
- **Ability to negotiate** – because in order to achieve targets you will need to negotiate both with clients and with other staff and agencies
- **Networking skills** – because you will need to cultivate contacts in order to find information, suppliers or services
- **In-depth knowledge** – because, depending on the job you are doing, you will need a detailed understanding of the sector you are working in, of local and national government policies and strategies relating to this sector and of the law which is relevant to your work.

WORKING WITH CHILDREN

If you work with children, it is particularly important that you have:

- The ability to communicate with young people in a way which is both effective and sensitive
- An understanding of the needs of children
- A knowledge of child development
- Lots of energy and patience – because working with children can be physically and mentally demanding.

Quiz

If you've read through all the qualities listed above and think you might fit the bill, try the quiz below – it's just a bit of fun, but it may help you decide if you're the sort of person who would suit a career in care. Answer the following multiple choice questions, then check out the answers to see how you did.

1. You see a three-year-old child out on the street and you can't identify who the child is with. Do you ...

   A. Go up to the child and ask where their parent/carer is and make sure they are safe?
   B. Get on with what you're doing – after all, your life is more important?
   C. Tut to yourself, tell the child off for not staying with their parent/carer and then go about your business?

2. You're on a very full train and all the seats are taken. A young father carrying his toddler gets on at the next stop. Do you ...

   A. Look out of the window and pretend you haven't seen them?
   B. Offer him your seat – it wouldn't be safe for him to stand on the train carrying a toddler?
   C. Ask the person sitting next to you to offer up their seat, as you've been on your feet all day and your legs are aching?

3. You're waiting at a bus stop and an older lady starts talking to you. Do you ...

   A. Nod politely and then turn away – you don't want to get involved?
   B. Pretend you haven't heard and pretend you're looking for something in your bag?
   C. Chat with the older lady – she may be lonely and not have spoken to anyone all day?

4. You pass a woman pushing a man who is a wheelchair user as you're walking up the street. The wheelchair user drops his glove on the floor, but doesn't notice. Do you ...

   A. Pick it up and hand it to the wheelchair user?
   B. Pick it up and hand it to the person pushing the man in the wheelchair?
   C. Ignore it – it's not your glove so why should you care?

5. You see a job advertised as a care assistant and note that you will be required to undergo training while you work. Do you ...

   A. Apply – you really want the job, and you want to be able to do the job to the best of your ability with the new skills the training provides?
   B. Not apply – you were interested in the job, but having to train and gain qualifications puts you off?
   C. Apply – you are happy to do the training, because this job will be a stepping stone to progress and develop to become a team leader or a manager?

6. You've just left school and you're considering a career in social care. Do you ...

   A. Look around for a job in social care – you'll soon find out whether you like it or not?
   B. Do some volunteer work to find out whether the social care sector is really for you?
   C. Speak to someone working in the social care sector who would be able to tell you all about it and give you some contacts?

7. You've got a job as a care assistant, but you really want to travel. What do you do?

   A. Hand in your notice at work and go and travel – you'll think about your career when you've run out of money.
   B. Consider working as a care volunteer abroad in countries that really need your help.
   C. Forget travelling – it was just an impossible dream anyway.

8. A job is going as a support worker. Which of the following candidates do you think is most likely to get the job?

   A. Sadie – she is 18, and has just spent four years caring for her grandmother at home.
   B. Paresh – he has just come back from Guatemala where he was a volunteer in an education programme.
   C. Gemma – she was previously a nurse and she wants to get back into work now that her children have started school.

9. One of your friends mentions that they are thinking of working in the care sector but mentions that she doesn't want to work long hours, she wants a job that she can forget about when she leaves work and she has a lot of personal problems at the moment, so she doesn't really have any time for anyone else's. Do you think that a job in care is the right thing for your friend?

A. Yes, definitely.
B. No, absolutely not.
C. Not at the moment. She needs to sort out her problems so she can deal with other people's needs and be prepared to put her own aside while she is at work.

10. Which of the following best describes your personality?

A. You're patient, tolerant and diplomatic.
B. You're bubbly, you have loads of energy and a good sense of humour and you know how to make people smile.
C. You're fairly shy, but considerate and a good listener.
D. You like things your own way and lose your fuse if you don't get it.
E. None of the above.

ANSWERS

1. **A.** Making sure that the child is safe shows that you have a sense of social responsibility and that you care about other people's welfare – these are very important values for care workers. If you picked **C** then you did show some concern, which is good – but you pre-judged the situation and did not

ensure that the child was safe, which is not very responsible. If you chose **B** then this suggests that you care more about yourself than the welfare of other people who are more vulnerable than you, and therefore you may not be ideally suited to a career in care.

2. **B**. Offering your seat shows that you were concerned about the safety of the child and that you realised that somebody carrying a young child deserved a seat more than you did – again this shows a sense of social responsibility and sensitivity to the needs of those around you, and suggests that you may have an aptitude for a caring role. If you chose **A** or **C** then you may not have the considerate attitude required by a caring career.

3. **C**. Chatting to the lady shows you have patience and are a good listener and communicator – again these are important skills for care. If you chose **A** or **B** then you may find it hard to make an effort for other people. It doesn't cost anything to offer a bit of conversation to an old lady at a bus stop; she may well live on her own and not talk to anybody all day – you need to learn to think about things from the point of view of those you are caring for.

4. **A**. Handing the glove to the wheelchair user shows both that you have a caring attitude and that you are not prejudiced, because you treated the wheelchair user as an individual. If you picked **B** (handing the glove to the person pushing the man) then you may have a caring attitude but you need to develop a more open mind towards people and not judge them on stereotypes. (For a detailed look at prejudice and how to overcome it, see *Real Life Issues: Prejudice*, published by Trotman). If you chose **C** then you

will have to seriously reconsider your attitudes if you want to work in the care sector.

5. **A** or **C**. Training and qualifications are key aspects of work in the care sector and you need to recognise the importance of gaining new skills in order to progress and develop and to make sure you do your job to the best of your ability. If you picked **B** then you will have to consider an alternative career, because training is compulsory for all care staff.

6. Any of these answers is good, but if you chose **B** or **C** it really shows that you are doing your research in order to get as much experience as possible before embarking on your career. This is extremely important, as a career in care is not for everyone. Voluntary work is a particularly good way to test the water – see page 48 for more information on how to get volunteering experience.

7. **B**. Care is a good career choice for those who want to travel as there are many volunteering opportunities abroad. Not only will you get to see other parts of the world and gain valuable work experience, but you will also be playing a major part in helping vulnerable people.

8. All three of these candidates are potential employees because they've all got experience of caring for other people. Remember, caring for members of your family counts!

9. **C**. Now is probably not the right time for your friend to take on a care job. If she has a lot of personal problems she should probably sort them out first – working in care can be mentally challenging and it takes a particularly strong person to cope with this alongside their own personal issues

(although it is possible!). It is very likely that your friend will have to work nightshifts or weekends, so she needs to take time to think about whether she is willing to do this. On the other hand, if your friend is really set on care as a career, she should not give up on it; she could work in a more administrative role until she has worked through her personal problems and feels ready to deal with other people's.

10. **A, B** or **C**. All three of these personality types can make successful carers. If you chose **D** or **E** then you probably have the wrong kind of temperament for a job of this nature. You have to do what's best for other people's needs and as you work in a team these decisions have to be made jointly, so you're not always going to get your way.

FINDING OUT MORE ...

So, how did you get on? By now you should have a clearer idea of whether you are suited to a career in care. If you are, great! Now you need to do some serious research. The previous chapters should have given you an idea of the kind of area you would like to work in; you need to find out as much as you can about the jobs that interest you so that you can target your job applications and/or training in the right direction.

The Resources section at the end of the book contains loads of useful websites and organisations that can offer detailed information and, as mentioned above, talking to people already working in the sector can be very helpful. However, the best way to find out about working in care and to make sure it's really for you is to get some experience. Volunteering is an excellent way to do this.

VOLUNTEERING

Volunteering is a good way to start off any career, and the care sector is no exception. Not only will volunteering develop your skills, knowledge and understanding of care work, but it may even open the door to your first job. It's also the best way to find out if working in care really is what you want to do. If it's not, then no harm done – but if it is, then the personal experience gained will be great for your career prospects and to add to your CV.

IN THE UK

There are various organisations that you can contact to get volunteer work. Try the ones below (see the Resources section at the end of this book for contact details):

- Community Service Volunteers (CSV)
- Millennium Volunteers – if you are aged between 16 and 24
- Volunteering England
- Citizens Advice Bureau (CAB)
- Your local Social Services Department – see http://local.direct.gov.uk/mycouncil to find your nearest council
- Your local paper.

Not only will volunteering develop your skills, knowledge and understanding of care work, but it may even open the door to your first job.

ABROAD

One of the great things about working in care is that your skills are always needed abroad. If you want to combine work and travel, what better way than to use your skills to benefit people in developing countries. Gaining experience of working overseas can be both rewarding and life-changing. It can also rejuvenate your passion for why you chose to work in care in the first place.

Organisations such as Voluntary Service Overseas (www.vso.org.uk) always have a demand for qualified, registered and experienced care workers, particularly those with managerial or training experience. VSO recruits volunteers and organises their return flights, insurance, national insurance, living allowance and accommodation. Most placements are for two years. Contact VSO for further details.

There are also other organisations that place volunteers, but you may need to pay for their services, as well as for other expenses including your flights. Placements vary in length from six weeks to 12 months or longer. Here are a few:

● Challenges Worldwide
● Gap Guru
● International Voluntary Service
● UN Volunteers
● WorldWide Volunteering.

See the Resources section at the end of this book for contact details. Some employers make it possible to take a career break plan which entitles you to unpaid leave to undertake volunteer work. More detailed information on volunteering is available in *Charity and Voluntary Work Uncovered*, published by Trotman.

LAURA TOWERS

Case study 2

SUPPORT WORKER

*Laura is a support worker at a Mencap
residential home for people with learning
disabilities, where she has been working
for the last two years.*

'I provide support to people with a learning
disability and help them to lead
independent and fulfilling lives. I help
people to cook and clean within their
home, offer support with personal care and
medication needs and help them manage
their finances. I also encourage and help
residents to lead an active life with college,
work placements and a wide range of
leisure activities. We provide 24-hour care
and support for the residents within their
homes.

'This job is completely different from what I
have done before. I fancied a change and
felt it would be an interesting job working
with people with learning disabilities. I was
particularly interested in working with
people with autism.

'To do my job you don't need any
particular qualifications, as long as you
have the right values and attitudes, treat

It is a
rewarding
and fulfilling
job and
every day is
different,
added to
which you
are constant
learning.

people as individuals, common sense and willingness to learn. There is a national Diploma in Care that would be useful, but it is not essential as Mencap have an in-house training programme.

'I had no training or experience with people with learning disabilities when I started this job. Mencap have a training programme. You start with a six-week induction course which involves working through modules and attending courses that relate to them such as first aid, moving and handling, health and safety and hygiene. When the induction course is completed you move on to the Mencap Foundation course which takes six months. Again you work through the modules and attend courses relating to those modules such as protection from abuse, positive approach, communicating and valuing people. After completing these programmes, all staff are then expected to study for NVQ level 2 or 3. Members of staff are regularly sent on training courses on subjects such as autism, epilepsy, diabetic training, diversity awareness, self-defence, active support and protecting vulnerable adults, which are all very interesting and useful.

To do my job you don't need any particular qualifications, as long as you have the right values and attitudes, treat people as individuals, common sense and willingness to learn.

'It is a rewarding and fulfilling job and every day is different, added to which you are constantly learning. It is good to be able to make a difference in people's lives, and it's great to be able to organise day trips out that relate to their interests, such as trips to the theatre, gigs, museums, galleries and wildlife parks, and see them enjoying themselves.

'The hours are very long and it can be extremely mentally demanding. There is a risk of violence, especially with the autistic residents. There is also an awful lot of paperwork such as risk assessments, daily reports, incident reports and health and hygiene reports.

'I would encourage anyone into support work if they have an interest in people, energy, enthusiasm and the urge to do something worthwhile and different. But I would also warn them of the long hours and the mentally demanding nature of the job – because of this, it is not the best job to be in if you have ongoing problems in your personal life.'

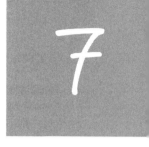

Training day

To help you decide which area of the care sector might be of interest to you, it's important to get an idea of the qualifications and training you might need. As care becomes increasingly recognised as a professional industry, the government has ensured that gaining skills and qualifications of a national standard has become a requirement. In April 2002, the Care Standards Act was implemented, meaning that all care staff must be trained and qualified to a nationally recognised standard.

You can start a job in care without qualifications, but you will be expected to join in a programme of 'continuous

---

A DRAMATIC QUALIFICATIONS TURNAROUND

Prior to 2002, 80% of the social care workforce had few or no qualifications at all. However, a 2004 survey carried out by the Office for National Statistics revealed that 89% of social care workers now hold qualifications. The percentage of workers with qualifications at each level breaks down as follows:

- Level 1: 20%
- Level 2: 29%
- Level 3: 14%
- Level 4: 23%
- Level 5: 3%.

professional development', which means you will be sent on courses, or train on the job to learn the necessary skills and progress. However, some jobs in the care sector, such as social worker or occupational therapist, will require you to have qualifications before you enter. This chapter will take you through what is required for each work area.

SOCIAL CARE

You can access most entry-level social care jobs (such as care assistant or personal assistant) without any formal qualifications. Once you start work you will be given training as outlined below.

INDUCTION AND FOUNDATION TRAINING

Induction training is provided by all employers during your first six weeks of employment to make sure that you are 'fit to practice'. This is followed by foundation training, which lasts a further six months and is mostly supervised by your manager at work. Once you have completed these two stages you can become professionally recognised, and you can use the work you have done to count towards a National Vocational Qualification in Health and Social Care (see below).

NATIONAL VOCATIONAL QUALIFICATIONS (NVQs)

NVQs (or Scottish Vocational Qualifications – SVQs) are work-based qualifications recognised throughout the UK. Detailed information on NVQs is available on the QCA website (www.qca.org.uk), but here are a few key points:

- NVQs are evidence that you are competent to do your job and that you understand the reasoning behind the tasks you carry out. They are based on National Occupational

Standards set up by the Skills for Care and Development Sector Skills Council – see www.topssengland.net for more information.

- NVQs are made up of a number of units of competence
- The full NVQ is gained when the set number of units from a range of choices has been achieved
- You are assessed for your NVQs while you work – there are no exams
- NVQs are available at different levels (1-5) and in different subjects depending on your job area and responsibilities, right up to management level
- NVQs are available to full-time, part-time, paid and voluntary social care workers
- The time taken to complete your NVQ is flexible – there is no time limit. They normally take between nine and 24 months to complete, though on average they take a year
- Funding of NVQs may be from your employer or from the Learning and Skills Council.
- NVQs are mainly awarded by the following bodies: City and Guilds, Edexcel, CACHE (Council for Awards in Children's Education), SQA, Oxford Cambridge and RSA. See the Resources section at the end of this book for contact details of each organisation.

NVQs relevant to work in social care are:

- Health and Social Care, available at levels 2, 3 and 4 (at levels 3 and 4, you can choose to specialise in care for adults or for children and young people)
- Registered Managers Award (Adult), available at level 4
- Managers in Residential Childcare Award, available at level 4.

Skills that you will learn as a new entrant which will lead to your NVQ levels 2 and 3 in Health and Social Care include:

- Hygiene
- Health and safety
- Lifting techniques
- Interpersonal skills for dealing with patients and their families.

Your employer will advise you on which NVQ to take and help you with the registration process.

APPRENTICESHIPS

The Apprenticeship initiative in Health and Social Care is an NVQ-based programme with additional elements to enhance the NVQ. It includes an NVQ level 2 and Advanced Apprenticeships at level 3. The work-based Apprenticeship programme is for young people aged between 16 and 24. If you would like to find out more about the Apprenticeship scheme then contact Skills for Care or your local Learning Skills Council (see the Resources section at the end of this book).

COMMUNICATION SUPPORT WORK

If you want to work as a communication support worker with deaf people you may need to work towards some or all of the Council for the Advancement of Communication with Deaf People (CACDP) certificates listed below:

- Certificate in British Sign Language, level 2
- Certificate in Note-taking for Deaf People, level 2
- Certificate in Electronic Note-taking for Deaf People, level 2

- Certificate in Lipspeaking, level 3
- Certificate in Communication and Guiding Skills with Deaf/blind people, level 3.

The National Association for the Tertiary Education of Deaf People (NATED) should be able to provide you with further information. NVQs at levels 3 and 4 are also available in British Sign Language.

The RNIB (Royal National Institute for the Blind) also run courses for teaching assistants in awareness of issues affecting people who are blind or have visual impairments.

FAMILY SUPPORT WORK

Like most areas of social care work, you can get a job as a family support worker without any formal qualifications and, as you work, gain NVQ qualifications in Health and Social Care or Children's Care, as well as a CACHE Diploma in Childcare. You could then move on to take a foundation degree in Professional Studies in Family Support and even, eventually, a postgraduate degree in Child Protection and Family Support.

SOCIAL WORK

Social Workers must gain a professional **Social Work degree** in order to practice. The degree takes three years to complete full-time, but it can be studied part-time or via distance learning. Graduate entrants or mature students with the relevant experience may take less time to qualify. As a social work student you will spend 200 days on practice work, enabling you to build up the experience you need when you begin employment.

ENTRY REQUIREMENTS

In order to get a place on a Social Work degree course, you will need to have Key Skills level 2 in English (which is the equivalent to a GCSE grade C). You will also need one of the following:

- At least 2 A levels (or equivalent)
- NVQs in Health and Social Care and/or relevant work experience within the care sector.

It is advisable to get some voluntary experience in care-related work as this will increase your chances of being accepted onto a course.

FUNDING YOUR DEGREE

You may find that you are eligible for funding from your employer. However, if not, you will have your tuition fees paid and you may also be entitled to a bursary of up to £2900 a year and £500 towards placement costs. The bursary is not means-tested, and is available to those studying for a Social Work degree who fulfil the entry criteria – see www.gscc.org.uk for more information. You must normally also be resident in England.

MOVING UP ...

Once you have qualified, you need to register with the **General Social Care Council** – see www.gscc.org.uk for more information. You can go on to take an MSc in Advanced Social Work to develop your career further.

OCCUPATIONAL THERAPY

There are no formal entry requirements for occupational therapy support workers. However, some employers may require NVQs in Health and Social Care, and many will encourage you to study for these qualifications as you work.

To practice as an occupational therapist you need to be registered with the Health Professions Council as a qualified occupational therapist. In order to register you need to take a pre-registration programme in occupational therapy – these are usually in the form of a degree course lasting three years (although if you already have a degree, you may be able to follow an accelerated course). Funding is usually available either from your employer or via a bursary – see www.cot.org.uk for more information.

COUNSELLING

Although in theory anyone can set themselves up as a counsellor, you will, in reality, and if you're serious about becoming one, need qualifications – preferably a degree, especially as this is a competitive job area.

In order to gain paid work, most counsellors are accredited by a reputable organisation – this provides their clients with a guarantee that they have undertaken suitable training and will provide a professional service by following a code of ethics and practices. Accreditation is gained via completion of a recognised counselling course, which will involve supervised counselling practice. The main organisations offering accreditation are the British Association for Counselling and Psychotherapy (BACP) and the United Kingdom Council for Psychotherapy (UKCP).

You may find that you need to be at least 21 to enrol on a counselling course, as age is considered a positive advantage in this kind of work. Courses available range from brief evening classes to postgraduate diplomas and degrees. Some employers will offer training programmes for counsellors.

WORKING WITH CHILDREN

There are no formal qualifications required for care work with children, but some employers may ask for qualifications and you may also wish to undertake training to enhance your career prospects and gain promotion. Courses you could undertake include:

- CACHE Certificate and Diploma in Childcare and Education (specialises in working with babies, children with individual needs and children under 8)
- CACHE and National Childminding Association's Diploma in Home-based Childcare, available at level 3 (specialises in working with children from birth to 16)
- BTEC National Qualification in Early Years, Working with Children or Teaching/Classroom Assistant
- BTEC Certificate for Teaching Assistants, available at levels 2 and 3
- NVQ in Children's Care, available at levels 2 and 3
- NVQ in Learning and Development, available at levels 2 and 3.

WHAT SUBJECTS SHOULD I TAKE AT SCHOOL?

'All this is very interesting', you may be thinking, 'but I'm still at school, and most of the training mentioned in this chapter takes place either at university or in the workplace – so what can I do *now*?'. If you are still at school and intend to follow a career in care then there are relevant qualifications to prepare you for entry to work. Here are some of the possibilities you could look at:

- **GCSEs**: The GCSE in Health and Social Care (Double Award) will give you a good foundation in the subject and can be used to access level 3 study when you leave.
- **A level**: The A level in Health and Social Care (previously a VCE) is offered by AQA, Edexcel and OCR and is available either as a single or a double award. It is a level 3 qualification and therefore equivalent to the level 3 NVQ.
- **BTEC**: There are a number of BTEC Awards, Certificates and Diplomas available in Health and Social Care, ranging from level 1 through to level 4. Some of these may be offered by your school or local further education college, and they are also suitable for people no longer at school who wish to access employment in social care work.

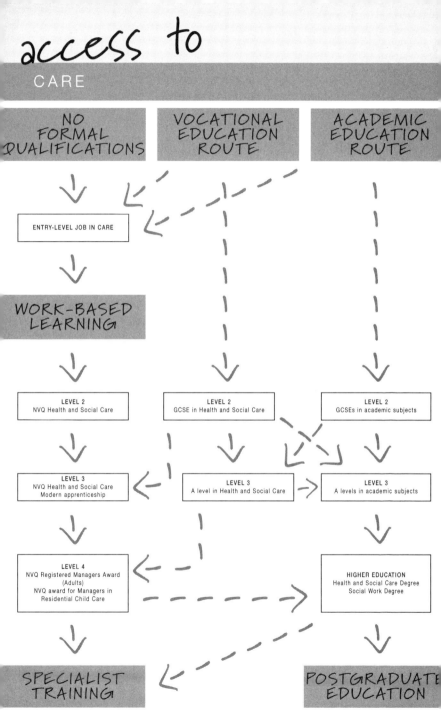

access to
CARE

NO FORMAL QUALIFICATIONS

VOCATIONAL EDUCATION ROUTE

ACADEMIC EDUCATION ROUTE

ENTRY-LEVEL JOB IN CARE

WORK-BASED LEARNING

LEVEL 2
NVQ Health and Social Care

LEVEL 2
GCSE in Health and Social Care

LEVEL 2
GCSEs in academic subjects

LEVEL 3
NVQ Health and Social Care
Modern apprenticeship

LEVEL 3
A level in Health and Social Care

LEVEL 3
A levels in academic subjects

LEVEL 4
NVQ Registered Managers Award (Adults)
NVQ award for Managers in Residential Child Care

HIGHER EDUCATION
Health and Social Care Degree
Social Work Degree

SPECIALIST TRAINING

POSTGRADUATE EDUCATION

PAULA ARMFIELD

Case study 3

SOCIAL WORKER

Paula is a social worker based in a child and family psychiatry unit. She has a Master's in Clinical Social Work from Boston College Graduate School of Social Work.

'To do a job like mine you need experience – ideally of child protection and family support work, of working with looked-after children in foster care and residential placements and of needs assessments and local authorities. You also need knowledge of child development, the Children's Act, Department of Health guidelines and regulations, patterns of family life, research in childcare, child protection and family support and the ability to work with families in a sensitive and empowering way. I work as part of a multidisciplinary team which provides clinical work – ie parenting skills training, family therapy, etc. I could go on ...

'The advantages of my work are that I have shared responsibility and that I get to think around complex cases (although this can also be a downside at times!). The children we see are those that the

The advantages of my work are that I have shared responsibility and that I get to think around complex cases (although this can also be a downside at times!).

outpatient teams do not feel they can get a 'handle' on. For example, the child may have a serious psychiatric disorder which requires five-day inpatient treatment. This is good because we can help make a difference, but it can also be quite sad too.

'One of the downsides to my job is that although we can make very thorough assessments and provide intensive intervention, we know that what we recommend or feel the child or family may need might not be delivered by the services (education, psychiatric or social services) once the child leaves.

'If anyone is interested in becoming a social worker, then I would recommend visiting and talking to people to find out what options there are. Placements at ours or similar units are possible.'

Making up your mind

One way of working out whether care is the career for you is to look at all the advantages and disadvantages, and working out which side, to you, outweighs the other. Throughout this book and in the case studies, a number of pros and cons have been mentioned – to help you collect your thoughts together, they are all listed together in this chapter.

ADVANTAGES

- **Worthwhile and rewarding job** – at the end of the day you can go home knowing that you've made a difference to the quality of someone's life. Every day you will have the opportunity to bring about positive developments and progress (eg diverting and breaking the cycle of antisocial behaviour). If you can change the way someone lives their life for the better that can only be a positive thing for that person and for the community at large. What a wonderful thing to achieve.
- **People** – you will get to meet new people, who you will spend time with and really get to know. Gaining their trust and building relationships with them can be extremely rewarding.
- **Teamwork** – you will share a common goal with your colleagues and with the outside agencies with whom you work. Working together towards a collective goal is

satisfying and you are much more likely to get positive results when you work as a team. You will also benefit from professional support from your colleagues.

- **Independence** – in care work you will always be part of a team, but some jobs (such as social work) give you the opportunity to manage your own time and make your own decisions. Having a sense of personal responsibility is good for you and your self-esteem.

- **Flexible hours** – from full-time to part-time and everything in between; you can find a shift pattern that suits your out-of-work commitments and lifestyle.

- **Variety** – every day is different, and variety, as we all know, is what makes a job interesting . Who wants the same old routine every day? Care careers also offer a wide range of different settings to work in – hospitals, day centres, private homes, in the community ...

- **Training** – you'll always be learning, and will have the opportunity to gain new skills and qualifications which will develop you in your work and as an individual. You can use these to get promotion or transfer them to another career if ever you decide you need a change.

- **Career prospects** – this is a growing sector and there are plenty of job opportunities. Once you are in, you should be able to gain promotion and/or to move into more specialised areas of the field corresponding with your particular interests. You might be a care assistant now, but you could be a fully qualified social worker in a few years time.

DISADVANTAGES

- **Emotional challenge** – working in care can be emotionally draining and mentally challenging – and it isn't generally the easiest job to switch off from when you go home, particularly if things aren't going to plan. At times you may feel upset and exhausted. Dealing with ignorance and prejudice and stigma can make your job even harder.

- **Physical challenge** – care work can be physically strenuous, especially if it involves a lot of lifting or carrying. You can come home feeling completely exhausted if you don't ensure you keep fit.
- **Lack of power** – you may have a lot of responsibility, but not the power to make decisions. This can be hugely frustrating if you can see the right solution, but no one else can. Similarly, although it is good to work as a team with other organisations, you can't control what the other organisations do and sometimes communication breakdown can lead to frustrating delays which you can't prevent.
- **Stress** – to add to the emotional strain, the consequences of getting it wrong can be very upsetting, both to you and to the other people concerned, which can be stressful. You may also be under pressure to produce reports and briefings to short deadlines.
- **Wages** – the staring salary isn't always as great as in comparable jobs and you may have to work for a while before you benefit from a better wage.
- **Funding** – you may have to apply for funding for a case you are working on – this is time consuming and the end result uncertain. It can be distressing if, for example, you can't recruit enough carers to foster children or young adults who may have complex needs, or if funding doesn't come through for a project you've put a lot of time and energy into
- **Working hours** – although in theory you should have some control over the hours you work, you may

sometimes find yourself working very long or unsociable hours and therefore perhaps missing out on extracurricular events or being out of sync with other members or your family or friends.

● **Paperwork** – this can drive you mad, especially when you feel you have more important things to be getting on with.

Consider each point in the lists above carefully – you could even try giving each one a mark out of ten to show how important you think it is, then add up the totals on each side; this may help you weigh up how you feel. Of course, whatever you decide will depend on factors that are important to you.

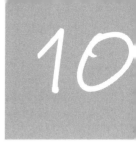

Career opportunities

Now that you've looked at the different areas of the care sector, found out about the training, looked at the pros and cons and decided that it's still the career you want to pursue, it's time to look to the future.

MAKING CARE YOUR CAREER

First of all, you need to think about what kind of care work you would like to make your career. Try asking yourself the following questions:

- Who do you want to care for? Do you want to work with children and families, older people, people with disabilities, people with mental health issues, people who have long-term illnesses, young offenders or people with substance abuse problems... ? Or don't you mind who you are working with as long as you are helping someone?
- What kind of environment would you like to work in? Do you want to work in a hospital, in a care home, in people's

private homes or out and about in the community? Would you like to work in the private or the public sector?

Chapter 3 gives an explanation of the different kinds of jobs available – which ones correspond with the kind of work you would like to do? Once you've decided on that, you need to work out what level you would like to enter at. Try asking yourself the following questions:

- Are you happy to start your career as a care assistant or a home care worker and work up, or do you want to become a social worker right from the outset?
- Are you better suited to work-based training, or should you go to college or university and do a degree?

Have a look at Chapter 7 to remind you of the training options available. Think about the different routes you can take to achieve your dream job and decide which is the best approach for you.

And once you've got that first job, where might your career take you? Remember, you can work your way up the NVQ framework; the higher-level NVQ qualifications (combined with the experience you will be gaining as you work in the sector) should enhance your promotion prospects and enable you to gain more senior positions.

Of course, once you've gained your NVQs, you can go on to do further qualifications.

DID YOU KNOW?

There are approximately 1.18 million care workers in Great Britain, comprising social care workers and childcare workers as well as managers and administrative staff.

Source: Office for National Statistics

It is possible to enter a career in social care with few or no relevant qualifications and work your way up into a management position or study for a degree, then move into social work. The diagram below should give you an overview of the options available at each level, and where they may lead.

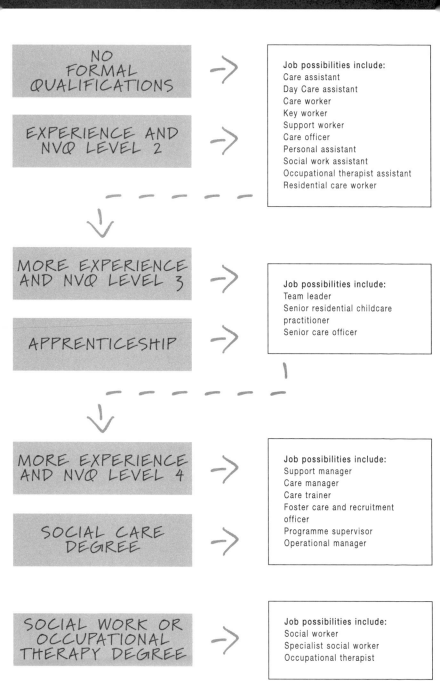

NO FORMAL QUALIFICATIONS

EXPERIENCE AND NVQ LEVEL 2

Job possibilities include:
Care assistant
Day Care assistant
Care worker
Key worker
Support worker
Care officer
Personal assistant
Social work assistant
Occupational therapist assistant
Residential care worker

MORE EXPERIENCE AND NVQ LEVEL 3

APPRENTICESHIP

Job possibilities include:
Team leader
Senior residential childcare practitioner
Senior care officer

MORE EXPERIENCE AND NVQ LEVEL 4

SOCIAL CARE DEGREE

Job possibilities include:
Support manager
Care manager
Care trainer
Foster care and recruitment officer
Programme supervisor
Operational manager

SOCIAL WORK OR OCCUPATIONAL THERAPY DEGREE

Job possibilities include:
Social worker
Specialist social worker
Occupational therapist

Case study 4

ART TUTOR

Lynn Towers has been an art tutor for people with mental health issues for four years, the first one of which was voluntary. She has a C&G Stage 1 in Further Education.

'I was already interested in art and had a friend suffering from mental health issues which led me to become interested in 'outsider art' as a consequence.

'I work with a group of students with varying mental health issues and teach them art (ie drawing and painting) from scratch. I design my own classes to suit the experience and abilities of the learners. Some of my students won't have picked up a paint brush since school. I am interested in the group dynamic and build up the confidence of the learners through reassurance and encouragement.

'I find my job very fulfilling and also inspiring in regard to my interest in outsider art. I also get a lot of enjoyment from helping my students to achieve their potential and seeing their confidence grow, both artistically and personally.

I get a lot of enjoyment from helping my students to achieve their potential and seeing their confidence grow, both artistically and personally.

'On the downside, the unpredictable behaviours of some of
the learners with severe mental health issues can be difficult.
In these circumstances I have to get their key workers and
other staff to assist. There is also too much paperwork,
which doesn't always feel necessary, and lack of funding
means that classes become shorter.

'I would advise anybody thinking of doing a job such as
mine to volunteer in the mental health system to see if they
have the aptitude for it – even if this only means two or three
hours a week, it would be well worth it.

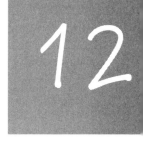

The last word

If you choose to work in care you will get tremendous satisfaction from seeing your clients' needs being met and your organisation develop for the good of the people it is working for. Choosing a career in care is a challenge, but tackling this challenge and getting good results is the most rewarding thing you can do. Are you going to make a difference to someone's life?

A GROWING SECTOR

The care sector is growing fast and there are plenty of opportunities for promotion if you fancy even more of a challenge. For example, the private sector has responded to the increase in demand for care services by opening new care homes (especially for older people), and this has brought about a growth in demand for registered care managers. Public care homes have been contracted out to independent organisations, which has had a similar effect. It's an exciting time to join this career area and there's probably a job out there that's just perfect for you – now all you have to do is go out there, find it and start making a difference!

DO YOU LIKE WORKING WITH PEOPLE?

☐ YES
☐ NO

ARE YOU AN EMPATHIC PERSON?

☐ YES
☐ NO

ARE YOU CONSIDERATE?

☐ YES
☐ NO

ARE YOU PATIENT?

☐ YES
☐ NO

DO YOU HAVE GOOD COMMUNICATION SKILLS?

☐ YES
☐ NO

DO YOU LIKE CHALLENGES?

☐ YES
☐ NO

ARE YOU WILLING TO UNDERTAKE WORK-BASED TRAINING?

☐ YES
☐ NO

ARE YOU PREPARED TO COPE WITH EMOTIONAL DEMANDS?

☐ YES
☐ NO

DO YOU WANT TO WORK IN A JOB THAT GIVES YOU VARIETY?

☐ YES
☐ NO

DO YOU WANT TO MAKE A DIFFERENCE TO PEOPLE'S LIVES?

☐ YES
☐ NO

If you answered 'YES' to all these questions then
CONGRATULATIONS! YOU'VE CHOSEN THE RIGHT CAREER!
Good luck, and well done for choosing to work in a profession that really makes a positive difference to the quality of people's lives.

If you answered 'NO' to any of these questions, then care may not be the career for you. However, you may like to consider some of the related occupations mentioned in Chapter 3, such as administrator, nursery nurse or charity fundraiser.

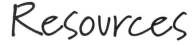

Resources

GENERAL

Care Ambassadors
Tel: 01305 010080
Website: www.careambassadors.info
A scheme to raise profile of careers in care and encourage young people into the profession.

Care Council for Wales
7th Floor
South Gate House
Wood Street
Cardiff CF10 1EW
Tel: 029 2022 6257
Website: www.ccwales.org.uk/careers

The Commission for Social Care Inspection (CSCI)
Tel: 0845 015 2255 (Minicom available on same number)
Email: enquiries@csci.gsi.gov.uk
Website: www.csci.org.uk
The CSCI inspect and report on care services to improve social care and stamp out bad practice.

Community Care
Community Care Magazine
Quadrant House
The Quadrant
Sutton
Surrey SM5 5AS
Tel: 020 8652 4861/4699

Website: www.community-care.co.uk
Website for everyone interested in care including news, jobs and discussion forum.

General Social Care Council
Golding's House
2 Hay's Lane
London SE1 2HB
Tel: 020 7397 5800 (Registration: 0845 070 0630)
Website: www.gscc.org.uk

Northern Ireland Social Care Council
7th Floor, Millennium House
Great Victoria Street
Belfast BT2 7AQ
Tel: 028 9041 7600
Website: www.niscc.info/careers

Scottish Social Services Council (SSSC)
Compass House
11 Riverside Drive
Dundee DD1 4NY
Tel: 0845 603 0891
Website: www.sssc.uk.com

Skills for Care and Development
Albion Court
5 Albion Place
Leeds LS1 6JL
Tel: 0113 245 1716
Website: www.topssengland.net

Social Care Association
Thornton House
Hook Road
Surbiton
Surrey KT6 5AN
Tel: 020 8397 1411
Email: web@scaed.demon.co.uk
Website: www.socialcaring.co.uk
The professional association for all those involved in care.

COUNSELLING

British Association for Counselling and Psychotherapy (BACP)
BACP House
35-37 Albert Street
Rugby
Warwickshire CV21 2SG
Tel: 0870 443 5252
Website: www.bacp.co.uk

Confederation of Scottish Counselling Agencies (COSCA)
18 Viewfield Street
Stirling FK8 1UA
Tel: 01786 475140
Website: www.cosca.org.uk

OCCUPATIONAL THERAPY

British Association of Occupational Therapists/College of Occupational Therapists
106-114 Borough High Street
Southwark
London SE1 1LB
Tel: 020 7357 6480
Website: www.cot.co.uk
Professional body for OT staff in the UK.

SPECIAL NEEDS

Council for the Advancement of Communication with Deaf People (CACDP)
Durham University Science Park
Block 4
Stockton Road
Durham DH1 3UZ
Tel: 0191 383 1155 (Textphone: 0191 383 7915)
Website: www.cacdp.org.uk

National Association for Special Educational Needs (NASEN)
NASEN House
4–5 Amber Business Village
Amber Close
Amington
Tamworth
Shropshire B77 4RP
Tel: 01827 311500
Website: www.nasen.org.uk

RNIB (Royal National Institute of the Blind)
105 Judd Street
London WC1H 9NE
Tel: 020 7388 1266
Website: www.rnib.org.uk

CHILDREN AND YOUNG PEOPLE

DFES Children's Workforce: Qualifications
Tel: 0870 000 2288
Website: www.dfes.gov.uk/childrenswfqualifications

Makaton Vocabulary Development Project
31 Firwood Drive
Camberley
Surrey GU15 3QD
Tel: 01276 61390
Website: www.makaton.org

National Childminding Association
Royal Court
81 Tweedy Road
Bromley
Kent BR1 1TG
Tel: 0845 880 0044
Website: www.pat.org.uk

Teachernet
Tel: 0870 000 2288
Website: www.teachernet.gov.uk

The TDA (The Training and Development Agency for Schools)
Portland House
Bressenden Place
London SW1E 5TT
Tel: 0870 4960 123
Website: www.tda.gov.uk
Information on Higher Level Teaching Assistants.

TRAINING AND QUALIFICATIONS

Learning and Skills Council
National Office
Cheylesmore House
Quinton Road
Coventry CV1 2WT
Tel: 0870 900 6800
Email: info@lsc.gov.uk
Website: www.lsc.gov.uk
Plan and fund vocational education and training for everyone.

National Association for Tertiary Education for Deaf People (NATED)
161 Mount Pleasant
Southcrest
Redditch
Worcester B97 4JJ
Tel: 07768 865137
Website: www.nated.org.uk

NHS Learning and Development Service

Tel: 0800 0150 850

This service is for people already employed within the National Health Service who would like advice on ways to learn, develop or gain qualifications to make the most of their potential. The service is open 8am to 8pm from Monday to Friday and the calls are free and confidential.

Skills for Care

Albion Court
5 Albion Place
Leeds LS1 6JL
Tel: 0113 245 1716
Website: www.skillsforcare.org.uk

Skills for Health

2nd Floor, Goldsmiths House
Broad Plain
Bristol BS2 0JP
Tel: 0117 922 1155
Website: www.skillsforhealth.org.uk

NVQ Awarding Bodies

CACHE (Council for Awards in Children's Care and Education)

Tel: 01727 818616
Website: www.cache.org.uk

City and Guilds

Tel: 020 7294 2800
Website: www.city-and-guilds.co.uk

Edexcel
Tel: 0870 240 9800
Website: www.edexcel.org.uk

SQA
Tel: 0845 279 1000
Website: www.sqa.org.uk

CAREERS AND JOBHUNTING

Care and Health
Golden Cross House
4th Floor, 8 Duncannon Street
London WC2 4 JF
Tel: 0870 901 7773
Website: www.careandhealth.com

Compass
Tel: 01892 784804
Email: admin@compassjobsfair.co.uk
Website: www.compassjobsfair.com
Compass organises three job fairs each year specifically for those looking for work in social care or social work. At each fair, copies of Compass – the complete guide to careers in Social Work and Social Care *(normal price £13.95) are distributed.*

Connexions
Website: www.connexions.gov.uk

Guardian Jobs
Website: http://society.guardian.co.uk/socialcare
Careers advice, jobmatch and the internet guide which lists useful websites for specific care sectors.

Jobcentre Plus
Website: www.jobcentreplus.gov.uk
Look under Childcare/Health/Care.

Jobsgopublic
Website: www.jobsgopublic.com/socialcarecareers
*Social care vacancies listed from the official local
government job site as well as other public sector and not-
for-profit organisations.*

Local Government
Website: www.LGcareers.com and www.lgjobs.com
*Careers website has advice and information on UK local
government careers; jobs website has live job vacancies in
local government.*

NHS Careers
PO Box 376
Bristol BS99 3EY
Tel: 0845 606 0655
Website: www.nhscareers.nhs.uk
*Information on NHS careers, job posts and benefits of
working in the NHS.*

Social Care Careers
Helpline: 0845 604 6404
Website: www.socialcarecareers.co.uk
*The Department of Health's Social Care website for issues
and matters relating to social care work in England including
jobs, also links to Northern Ireland, Scotland and Wales.*

Social Work Careers
Helpline: 0845 604 6404
Website: www.socialworkcareers.co.uk
Department of Health's Social Work website for information regarding social work including course finder.

VOLUNTEERING (UK AND OVERSEAS)

Challenges Worldwide
Tel: 0845 200 0342
Website: www.challengesworldwide.com

Citizens Advice Bureau (CAB)
Hotline: 0845 1 264 264
Website: www.citizensadvice.org.uk
Volunteer recruitment and find your local CAB in the UK on this website.

Community Service Volunteers (CSV)
Tel: 0800 374 991
Website: www.csv.org.uk/socialhealthcare

Gap Guru
Tel: 0800 032 3350
Website: www.gapguru.com

International Voluntary Service
Website: www.ivs-gb.org.uk

Millennium Volunteers
Website: www.connexions.gov.uk and
www.millenniumvolunteers.gov.uk

UN Volunteers
Email: information@unvolunteers.org
Website: www.unv.org

Volunteer Development England
Tel: 0845 305 6979
Website: www.volunteeringengland.org.uk

Volunteering England
Tel: 0845 305 6979
Website: www.volunteering.org.uk

Voluntary Service Overseas (VSO)
Tel: 020 8780 7200
Website: www.vso.org.uk

WorldWide Volunteering
Tel: 01935 825588
Website: www.worldwidevolunteering.org.uk

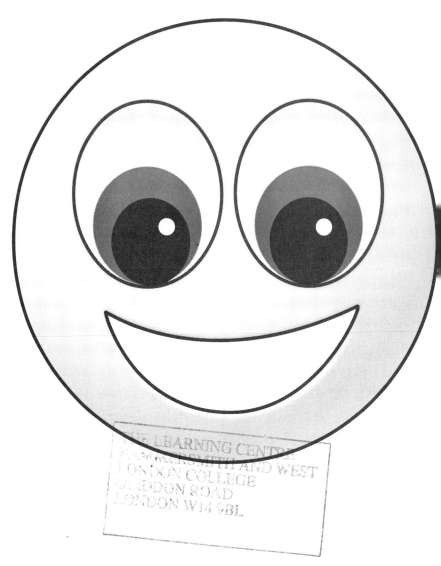

BE HAPPY

Eight out of the top ten happiest workers are vocational workers. City & Guilds has over 500 qualifications to choose from. You're just one click away from your future happiness.

CITYANDGUILDS.COM/HAPPY

City&
Guilds